Antioxidant

The natural way to fight cancer
And aging as well as reaching your
Optimum Health

Abagail Lewis

Contents

Introduction – What is an Antioxidant?

Chapter 1 – How do Antioxidants Work?

-Free Radicals

-The Antioxidants

Chapter 2 – What are the Best Antioxidants?

-Enzymatic and Non-Enzymatic

-Antioxidants Produced by the Body

-Antioxidants from Diet

Chapter 3 –The Benefits of an Antioxidant-Rich Diet

-Anti-Inflammatory

-Immune Benefits

-Anti-Aging

-Food Combinations

Chapter 4 – Antioxidants and Cancer

-Studies on Antioxidants and Cancer

-The Smoking Paradox

-The Conclusion

Chapter 5–Facts and Myths of Antioxidants

-FACT: Gene and DNA damage are both

implemented in Cancer and other Diseases

-MYTH: Taking Antioxidant Supplements Will

Prevent/Treat Cancer

-MAYBE: Antioxidants lessen the Effect of

Chemotherapy

-FACT: Tea is one of the best antioxidant sources

-MYTH: All vitamins are Antioxidants

-FACT: It is Impossible to have too Many

Antioxidants in Your Body

-MYTH: Superfoods are Important for an Antioxidant-Rich Diet

-FACT: Dietary Antioxidants are Superior

Chapter 6 – Antioxidants and Nutrition

-ORAC Values & Marketing

-Sports Nutrition

Chapter 7 – A Diet of Antioxidants

-Vegetables

-Fish:

-Fruits

-Grains

-Herbs

-Tea and Coffee

-Nuts

Conclusion

Introduction – What is an Antioxidant?

WITHIN THE LAST FEW YEARS, antioxidants have gotten a lot of press. Supposedly they fight cancer, Alzheimer's, aid weight loss, fight aging, and are a miracle substance that will cure every woe. In theory, the problem with this is it's not so realistic to believe that antioxidants will cure everything, but what is true is that science has shown antioxidants to be an effective combatant against many of the pollutants we face in modern life.

A hundred years ago cities dealt with coal smog, burning gas, and a few crazy (yet deadly) clothing dyes. Now you're less likely to die of arsenic poisoning from your dress but you're also being exposed to an enormous amount of chemical pollutants.

Many of these pollutants form free radicals in the body or cause the body to produce more through exposure.

Free radicals are a Reactive Oxygen Species that have unbound oxygen molecules. They react with enzymes, proteins, lipids, and other molecules within the body. In large amounts, they can disrupt and damage the cells of the body as well as disrupt DNA through a process called oxidation. DNA and cell damage from oxidation is often the cause of chronic disease. The damage that cells experience is known as oxidative stress. Antioxidants help to stabilize free radicals and prevent this from happening.

Chances are you've heard of "superfoods". They've been pretty popular recently and the reason for this is that they're often rich in antioxidants. Diets that are low calorie and rich in fruits and vegetables often contain high levels of antioxidants too. When combined with a lower calorie diet research has shown they can even prolong life. It is theorized that this helps lower the level of oxidative stress on the body, however, not all foods are created equal.

Since there are a variety of different antioxidants they are all thought to work in different ways. For example, Vitamin E molecules found in antioxidants can alter metabolism. It certainly isn't a question of "if" antioxidants work, they do, but how does it benefit you?

Even if the disease fighting enzymes weren't enough, antioxidants have also been shown to have a profound effect on aging. Just by taking in enough antioxidants you can slow the aging process.

So, antioxidants fight cancer, slow aging, rev your metabolism and basically perform miracles. It would be understandable if you're thinking that one single enzyme can't possibly to all this, it can't be true. This potent little enzyme should be in everyone's diet if that's the case. But how exactly do they work?

Chapter 1 – How do Antioxidants Work?

BEFORE UNDERSTANDING ANTIOXIDANTS, you have to understand what they are fighting against. Plant-derived polyphenols, aka antioxidants, have the ability to neutralize other molecules that could potentially harm our bodies' cells and cause them to malfunction. These harmful molecules usually have a free, unpaired electron which is why they are so reactive. The body likes cells to be orderly and in pairs so an unbound electron is usually looking for something to pair up with. The problem is we don't want these harmful cells to pair up with ours because they're going to cause damage. These are called free radicals.

Free Radicals

Free radicals come from a variety of different sources. Sometimes they are a byproduct of our own body processes but usually, they are a reaction to outside pollutants such as cigarette some, UV radiation, air pollution, medications, and chemicals in our daily lives. Free radicals are highly reactive. Once the free radical forms it causes a domino effect by continuing to multiply by stealing electrons from other cells, damaging them in the process. The damaged cells may also turn into free radicals themselves and the process snowballs. This is called oxidative stress because the reaction is called oxidation and at this point the oxidative molecules outnumber the protective enzymes.

We need oxygen to survive, but the chemical that gives us life is also slowly killing us. Oxidation in our bodies is what rust is to an iron bar – it's nothing more than a chemical reaction but it damages the original chemical makeup. When a fresh cut apple turns brown, that's oxidation happening right in front of your eyes.

There are 5 different types of free radicals, they are mostly oxygen derived.

1. Superoxide ion (O): Oxygen as a single molecule has an extra electron, this radical is especially damaging to DNA and mitochondria though it can affect other molecules.

2. Radical Hydroxyl (OH): One of the most reactive radicals, this is formed when the molecule loses an oxygen (HO^2). It actually cannot be eliminated by enzyme reaction and must be forcibly broken apart by antioxidant molecules. The molecule can damage just about every organic molecule in the body including DNA, proteins, lipids and even carbohydrates.

3. Singlet Oxygen: Formed by the natural immune process this radical targets LDL specifically.

4. Hydrogen Peroxide (H^2O^2): While this chemical itself isn't a free radical it freely attaches to others because of its structure which aids in the domino effect.

5. Reactive Nitrogen Species (NO) (RNS): Usually found in the body as nitric acid.

These free radicals not only steal enzymes from other cells but they cause far more damage while doing it. They can alter the structure of DNA bases, interfere with maintenance, and disrupt DNA duplication. They can also physically rip a molecule or cell apart. This process has been linked to over 60 different diseases. For example, the oxidation of lipoproteins leads to atherogenesis which causes atherosclerosis and will eventually develop into cardiovascular problems. If cell DNA becomes damaged cells may begin to grow abnormally and this can become cancerous.

The antioxidants work in two different ways to stop this from happening.

The Antioxidants

Antioxidants are an enzyme produced by the body that often attaches to the unbound electron and stops it from interfering with other cells in the body. It does this by simply providing an extra electron for the free radical to be attracted to, and then attached. Once the free radical cell is attached it becomes harmless as the antioxidant does not form a free radical as other cells might. This process is called chain-breaking. Antioxidants also have the potential to break these same bonds, by letting the free radical attach to its own electron it can then breaking it down into smaller molecules and destroy it. This is the enzyme acting as a preventative since it prevents the chain of free radicals from forming.

Antioxidants stop the chain reaction from continuing, but they are also used up in the process which is why it is so important to continue to provide the body with a good source of them. Depending on which free radical and which antioxidant are involved certain body systems may be more or less at risk. Your body does have the ability to produce some of its own antioxidants, but not all of them. The problem is that as we age our ability to do so also decline so it's important to have a good source of them in your diet.

Chapter 2 – What are the Best Antioxidants?

As we've seen not all foods are created equal, while some may be rich in antioxidants others might only be rich in one kind. It's important to have a variety of antioxidants to make sure you are protected against all 5 of the different types of free radicals. The USDA created a tool that scores how rich in antioxidants certain foods are. This is called the ORAC score, meaning the Oxygen Radical Absorbency Capacity. The higher the score the food has the more powerful it is for combating the damage of free radicals. The problem is that many processed foods have a misleading ORAC score because the manufacturers stuff them with artificial antioxidants that are not necessarily as effective.

The largest classes of antioxidants are flavinoids, and there are over 5,000 that have been identified so far. Not all of them are bio-available however so many flavinoids need to be consumed with other enzymes and minerals so that the body is able to make use of them or they just won't get absorbed.

Enzymatic and Non-Enzymatic

When it comes to antioxidants found in food there are two main types: Enzymatic and Non-Enzymatic. Each deals with free radicals according to the two methods we've already mentioned.

Non-Enzymatic Antioxidants work by chain-breaking the free radical process. Some of the most common non-enzymatic antioxidants found are Vitamins C and E, carotenoids, plant polyphenols and glutathione. Antioxidant supplements are usually made of non-enzymatic antioxidants.

Note: While glutathione has been touted as the antioxidant of antioxidants it isn't something that you should rely on indiscriminately. Glutathione levels have been shown to elevate when exposed to certain toxins, so it's a lot more complicated than that. Much of the information you can find on this enzyme is so scientific that it's hard to follow. The TL:DR version is that although glutathione has been shown to have effects on sleep disorders, Parkinson's, Hashimoto's and some mental health issues it's not a cure.

Ezymatic Antioxidants, on the other hand, work to breakdown and remove free radicals. They are much more prevalent than non-enzymatic antioxidants and work by flushing oxidants out as water through a 2 step process – first by converting them into hydrogen peroxide and then water. The process also requires a variety of trace metals and is much more complicated than simply breaking the bonds of the free radical molecules. This type of antioxidant cannot be made into a supplement and can only be formed in the body. Antioxidants can also be broken down into both large and small molecule classification. The enzymatic antioxidants tend to be the larger. Often the Albumin found in the chemical make-up of enzymatic antioxidants acts as the sacrifice for the free radical to destroy in place of cell DNA.

Antioxidants Produced by the Body

While each type of antioxidant has its own benefit it is important that you get a variety of different ones in your diet. As mentioned, glutathione has been often called the "only" antioxidant you need. The fact is, that you really need a variety of several antioxidants to fully protect your cells from the damage of free radicals. Some of the antioxidants you'll hear about most are those that are produced in the body, but you'll still need to keep the intake constant since they will be constantly used up.

The three most common antioxidants produced in the body are Glutathione, Alpha-Lipoic Acid, and CoQ10 (Ubiquinone). As you age your body struggles to produce these and supplementation is often necessary.

Glutathione is a tripeptide molecule that is found in every cell in the body. It is unique in that it actually supports other antioxidant activity. Its main function is to protect the mitochondrial cells from damage but it also works on slowing down the aging process and against radiation. Glutathione can be found in curcumin, eggs, dairy, and grass-fed meat.

Alpha-Lipoic Acid (ALA) is an enzymatic antioxidant that can help to regenerate other antioxidants. It is also the only one that can work within the structure of the brain so it is essential for dealing with brain degeneration, such as that found in Alzheimer's. ALA has also been shown to improve insulin sensitivity, remove heavy metals from the body, and to reduce inflammation caused by faulty genes.

CoQ10, or Ubiquinone, is also used by every cell in the body. It needs to be converted or found in it's often marketed as Ubiquinol. It has been linked to improved energy, to reduce aging, improved blood pressure, and immune support. Until you're between 25-30 your body is very efficient at converting CoQ10 to Ubiquinol, however as you age the process can become less efficient so it's important to look for a supplement that is in this form rather than the Ubiquinone so the body doesn't have to work as hard.

Asides from these your diet should also contain a variety of antioxidants that are not found in the body.

Antioxidants from Diet

Reservatrol is one that you'll most often see listed on products claiming to have antioxidant powers. This is most often found in fruits with darker colors such as grapes, cocoa, and even red wine. Like ALA, it can also work in the brain, and has been called one of the most effective age fighters. It also works to lower blood pressure, inhibit cancer growth, improve blood flow, and to work as a preventative for Alzheimer's.

Carotenoids are actually a pigment; it's what makes many fruits and vegetables such vibrant colors. There are actually over 700 different carotenoids. They can be split into two groups Carotenes and Xanthophylls. Carotenes have no oxygen atoms in their molecular makeup. Two of the most well known are beta-carotene (found in orange carrots), and lycopene (found in red tomatoes). Xanthophylls do have an oxygen atom. Common xanthophylls include lutein, zeaxanthin, canthaxanthin, and astaxanthin. Zeaxanthin is actually the most commonly occurring carotenoid and is found in peppers, grapes, squash, kiwi, and oranges.

Although astaxanthin is technically a carotenoid it's worth considering as a group on its own. The reason for this is that it's a naturally occurring antioxidant produced by marine algae. When it becomes dehydrated the algae produces this enzyme to protect itself from UV radiation, when ingested it can produce the same enzyme for your skin cells. In fact, it is over 500 times more powerful than Vitamin E at combating singlet oxygen formed from UV radiation. Astaxanthin can also work in the brain and eyes, something most carotenoids cannot do. It is extremely powerful and also has wider benefits. These include protection from macular degeneration, Alzheimer's, MS, reducing the risk of cancer, improving cardiovascular health and reducing the symptoms of a variety of age-related diseases. However, like glutathione, it's also touted as a "cure all" simply because it's so powerful and should be considered accordingly.

Vitamin C has been used as a therapy drug for hundreds of years. In 1904, Linus Pauling used high dose vitamin C therapy to kill cancer cells. It's one of the oldest known antioxidants and is also one of the most flexible. It acts as an electron donor for the most part, but also helps to specifically protect lipids and proteins from free radical damage. Though you can find vitamin C in supplement form it usually isn't so bioavailable as that found within whole foods.

Vitamin E is actually 8 different compounds broken into 2 groups. Half are tocopherols and tocotrienols. Usually, a balanced diet will mean you have the range of molecules available however if you're only taking them in supplement form you're actually only taking in 1 out of the 8 depending on your supplement choice.

Chapter 3 – The Benefits of an Antioxidant-Rich Diet

WE'VE ESTABLISHED THAT ANTIOXIDANTS are great fighters in helping our body battle free radicals but is that really it? Even if you're not at genetic risk for many of the diseases caused by free radicals you can still benefit from having an antioxidant rich diet. The reason for this is that the interaction between antioxidants and the body goes far beyond just fighting free radicals. Getting your antioxidants from your food means you're often getting a greater variety and better bioavailability than that in supplement form. In fact, you might be selling yourself short if you're only relying on supplements.

Anti-Inflammatory

A study from 2012 by Harvard Medical School found that antioxidants can help prevent the oxidation of lipids. Lipids (or fats) often cause inflammation and this can be exacerbated by their oxidation. By dealing with fat oxidation, you're also going to see a small amount of weight-loss. Inflammation is often the body's response to injuries and dead cells, it's a necessary part of the healing process but it can also cause a lot of health issues if it goes beyond this. Asthma, some cancers, diabetes, and even mental illness have all been linked to inflammation in different organs. Fat cells also produce cytokines which attract these inflammatory cells and are also prone to interaction with free radicals. Studies have shown the polyphenols found in coffee and teas are most effective at dealing with these types of free radicals.

Immune Benefits

By dealing with free radicals in the body, we also get a boost to the immune system. Vitamins C and E, selenium, and polyphenols are all formed by the body's own processes but are also essential in dealing with highly reactive free radicals. They help by neutralizing them and can even boost the immune system in case of infection. Studies have also shown that vitamin C is also important in preventing and fighting cancers. In fact, it has been found to be especially important when it comes to preventing breast cancer.

Anti-Aging

Many of the common antioxidants have also been found to have anti-aging properties. They can have some effect on both brain, eye and skin cell degeneration. In 2008, a study showed that blueberry-rich diets helped to improve the brain's ability to function by establishing stronger connections between neurons and improved memory. CoQ10 and Vitamin E are both strong anti-aging antioxidants. The damage our skin get's from UV exposure is strongly linked to how badly it ages which is why antioxidants that deal with free radicals related to it are so important if you want your skin to continue to look young.

Food Combinations

As well as their rawest form antioxidants in different foods can also be combined to make super antioxidants. These are a combination which can pack a powerful punch. For example blueberry, strawberry, and spinach are thought to work together to inhibit an enzyme that is thought to affect the brain. This means that together they can act against depression, schizophrenia, and even autism. Berries are especially high in antioxidants and they're also easy to combine in this way. Many popular smoothie mixes rely on combining antioxidants to get the most powerful kick. Combining antioxidants and fiber also produces a synergistic effect.

Chapter 4 – Antioxidants and Cancer

ONE OF THE MOST PREVALENT BELIEFS about antioxidants is that they are a miracle cure against cancer. When Linus Pauling did his tests using Vitamin C it was thought that this would be the end of the disease. What has happened in the century since is the murky stuff of conspiracy theorists. While some will tell you that the pharmaceutical companies buried the research in order to make money – just look at the doctor in Texas being sued by them for treating patients with the same method successfully. Others will tell you that even if the enzymes in antioxidants are effective against cancer cells it doesn't necessarily mean the same results in the body where you have any number of variables present.

Studies on Antioxidants and Cancer

The problem with much of the research into the link between cancer and antioxidants is that most of the trials weren't long-term and they also weren't effective at proving antioxidants were a preventative for cancer. In fact, such a study even showed that among a study group cancer rates did not differ between those taking an antioxidant and those taking a placebo.

The SU.VI.MAX trial, however, showed that men had a reduction in cancer risk while women saw no effect when taking beta-carotene. The problem with this study is that men naturally have a lower level of blood beta-carotene. The same trial however also showed that women who had taken antioxidants (C, E, Selenium, Beta-carotene, and Zinc) were also at risk of a higher rate of skin cancer.

Selenium, on the other hand, showed a significant reduction in cancer size when used in a trial against skin cancer as well as lung, prostate, and colon cancers. However, those with a low base selenium level were also most affected so it could simply show that a selenium deficiency increases the risk of cancer.

You can see where a lot of the research can be seen as confusing.

The Smoking Paradox

In fact, a 2014 Swedish study showed that some cancer patients may actually risk making their disease worse with an increased antioxidant intake. The study centered on smokers and people who were at risk for lung cancer with the aim of proving that antioxidants would actually decrease tumors (similar to the Selenium study). The problem was that the antioxidants were found to accelerate the progression of cancer by short-circuiting the body's immune response to the malignant cells. Another study showed that Vitamin E and Acetylcysteine also increased the tumor growth for mice infected with lunch cancer. Researchers concluded that antioxidants directly increased the number and aggression of tumors by threefold!

The Conclusion

Overall it can safely be said that while antioxidants may have anti-cancer properties once a patient is diagnosed antioxidants may actually do more harm than good. The 9 most well-known studies failed to provide enough evidence that antioxidant supplements actually helped with cancer prevention; however, other studies have shown that diets rich in antioxidant-rich foods are related to a lower cancer risk. It's important to remember that new studies come out all the time and there may soon be a proven link but it doesn't exist yet. It is also possible that the fact that almost all studies relied on man-made supplements were the real reason that research failed. Diets that are rich in complex mixtures of antioxidants might be the key that is missing within these studies.

Chapter 5 – Facts and Myths of Antioxidants

FACT: Gene and DNA damage are both implemented in Cancer and other Diseases

Studies have shown time and time again that many degenerative diseases and cancers are caused by our own body processes going wrong. In fact, it's often substances created by our own bodies that contribute to cancer and its growth. The oxidation reaction is damaging to chemicals and other molecules so it's safe to assume that the same link exists in our own bodies. Antioxidants have been proven to be effective against oxidation, cell degeneration, and DNA damage. Despite the failure of studies to connect the link dietary antioxidants are the key to this and not supplementation. Many supplements fail to provide the full range of antioxidants needed or the correct combinations for the body to use them against oxidative damage.

MYTH: Taking Antioxidant Supplements Will Prevent/Treat Cancer

In theory, a high presence of antioxidants in the body should prevent cancer, but research has struggled to come to any significant affirmative of this. The fact is that when studies focus on populations that have diets rich in antioxidants the populations have far lower rates of most cancers in comparison to those whose diets don't. Studies have supported that antioxidant supplements may have some effect against very specific cancers but the rate is below 10% which could also account for other variables. In fact, the smoking study previously mentioned showed just how wrong this assumption can be. Antioxidants are known to actually worsen certain cancers so they are far from being a miracle cancer cure.

MAYBE: Antioxidants lessen the Effect of Chemotherapy

Some chemotherapy drugs have been linked to increased oxidation in the body. Many of the side effects of chemotherapy have been shown to lessen with an increased intake of antioxidants. The data isn't very strong yet and more studies are needed. However, there has also been links to decreased effectiveness for some chemotherapy drugs for patients taking an antioxidant supplement.

FACT: Tea is one of the best antioxidant sources

Although it's a myth that simply drinking tea will lengthen your lifespan tea does have a high level of antioxidants in it, especially flavinoids. Drinking tea is an easy way to boost your antioxidant intake without having to make a huge dietary change. Not all teas are created equal. Despite the fact that green tea, oolong tea, and black tea all come from the Camellia Sinensis plant it is the huge difference in processing that affects the level of antioxidants found in each blend. Tea does have almost 10 times the amount of antioxidants found in many foods though, and it's prevalence in the East where most Western dietary diseases are lower can be linked to the prevalence of tea drinking.

MYTH: All vitamins are Antioxidants

Of the tens of thousands of different antioxidants, only a few are actually vitamins. While C and E are some of the most well-known most are mineral or enzymes. Enzymatic antioxidants, for example, are rarely vitamins. Polyphenols, found in many fruits and vegetables, are also not vitamins despite being highly prevalent.

FACT: It is Impossible to have too Many Antioxidants in Your Body

We've seen that oxidative stress is the imbalance of antioxidants and free radicals, when there are too many free radicals and too few antioxidants your body is at risk for disease. In theory, if you overload your body with antioxidants it could trigger and immune response that would then damage the body's own ability to produce them. The amount needed for this would have to be incredibly high, even toxic, for this to actually happen.

MYTH: Superfoods are Important for an Antioxidant-Rich Diet

While superfoods have often been touted as being "antioxidant rich" cures they're not essentials in your diet. Just because you spent $20 on some goji berries it doesn't mean that you can't get the same antioxidants from a 39¢ kiwi. In essence, all fruits are super in their own way and as long as you're eating a variety of them you'll still be getting the same antioxidant benefits. Most superfoods simply have slightly higher densities of antioxidants than others of similar make-up. For example, blueberries are very rich in antioxidants but it just happens that açai berries are even higher. The only reason these specific berries are "super" is simply marketing. If you're trying to make sure you've got a diet rich in all the necessary antioxidants than the easiest advice is to eat by colors.

FACT: Dietary Antioxidants are Superior

While it is possible to get antioxidants from supplements it has been proven time and time again that supplements are not as powerful or as effective as a varied diet. The combination of antioxidants, fiber, and other minerals in food are key to prevent and fight off disease. These additional benefits are not found in a supplement which is why they may not be as effective in trials. To improve the level of antioxidants in your body you have to look at your food intake and adjust accordingly.

Chapter 6 – Antioxidants and Nutrition

MOST ANTIOXIDANTS ARE FOUND in fruits and vegetables and conveniently if you don't like one vegetable there's a good possibility there is something similar that has the same antioxidants in it. For example, if you can't stand kale or spinach choose broccoli instead. Instead of eating oranges, choose a mango. Most fruits and vegetables can be grouped by color. The food rainbow is an ideal way to make sure that you're getting the full variety of antioxidants in your diet.

ORAC Values & Marketing

We mentioned the ORAC value at the beginning of this book, many foods will tell you that they have high ORAC values but almost all of the processed foods that are worried about their ORAC value get it from additives and supplements, not from natural sources. As research has shown, supplements rarely provide levels needed to see true benefits so it's best to stay away from them. In 2012, several class-action lawsuits were filed because of companies promoting their products with statements referring to natural sources of antioxidants while the products themselves contained synthetics. Hershey's chocolate, for example, used the fact that cocoa is high in flavinol antioxidants as a marketing ploy yet the alkalization process their chocolate goes through also eliminates any flavinol content.

Similarly many foods will proclaim they are "antioxidant rich" just to get your attention. They may also be packed with excess sugar and chemical preservatives that nullify any benefits you're getting from the antioxidants. Though they may not necessarily be harmful they are also not helpful either. Most companies want to sell you a product, they want to profit from you, which is why you should never simply believe any claims on packaging. In fact, it's easier to simply eat a varied whole food diet if you're trying to boost your antioxidant intake.

Sports Nutrition

Diet is incredibly important for athletes, and in the same way, antioxidants are doubly important for those who do a lot of aerobic exercise. Aerobic exercises increase oxidation in the muscle tissue and also increase lipid peroxidation. Athletes are at greater risk of free radical damage to their body because they're putting it under greater oxidative stress through exercise. This isn't to say that exercise is bad, and that you won't experience oxidation if you don't exercise, but it does show a higher rate. The use of antioxidants as a sporting supplement is obviously controversial because of the potential for an unfair performance advantage. Antioxidants may improve performance by lowering the effects of oxidation on the muscles and lowering oxidative damage.

Studies have shown that certain antioxidant levels in the body are greatly affected by exercise. A study by

Sastre showed that glutathione levels were greatly affected while others showed that they were only slightly affected. Some tenuous links have been found between antioxidants and the ability to recover after exercise more quickly.

There is some debate about whether or not antioxidant supplements might even be a necessity of good sports nutrition. Most athletes' diets are high in protein and high in calorie, and though the quality of food is good they may be missing out on having enough variation due to avoiding foods that might have higher sugars like fruit.

Chapter 7 – A Diet of Antioxidants

IF YOU TRULY WANT THE BEST QUALITY of antioxidants in your diet you need to choose foods accordingly. We've mentioned eating the rainbow, try and imagine each food grouped into a color – oranges with apricots, spinach with kiwi, tomatoes with strawberries etc. The reason you need to do this is because most antioxidants show themselves in food as a strong vibrant color. This is true whether the food is grown on a tree, on land or even in the sea! Many popular drinks are also high in natural antioxidants. Try and avoid sugar as much as possible since it's often stuffed with free radicals and causes inflammation.

Vegetables

Most vegetables are loaded with phytochemicals that act as antioxidants, however, green vegetables are especially rich in them. Phytochemicals help to eliminate free radicals that are carcinogens and can also reduce inflammation in the body. As we've seen, not all vegetables are equal. Many enzymes can become denatured by the cooking process rendering them useless. In fact, many who choose a raw diet do so for just this reason. Juicing and smoothies are an ideal way to boost your raw vegetable count since they are often lower in fat or calories, and you can create perfect antioxidant combinations. Many sprouted vegetable seeds are also higher in antioxidants than their full-grown versions. For example, pea sprouts are actually higher in protein and antioxidants than fully grown peas. Sprouts are a great source of both antioxidants and vitamins. Many of the enzymes and minerals found in sprouts are key to having a healthy immune system.

Leafy Greens: Darker greens like kale, collard, and spinach are all high in nutrients and antioxidants. They are especially high in vitamins A, C, E and are nutrient dense in calcium, magnesium, and potassium. Green vegetables are also high in the phytochemical kaempferol which has been studied for its cancer-fighting properties. Lettuce isn't as dense of a green vegetable but it does also have lutein and quercetin which are both important antioxidants. Frozen, chopped spinach is an ideal way to get extra greens in your diet as it can be mixed into smoothies, dips, and soups.

Artichoke: Artichokes have around 7,904 antioxidants per serving which makes them one of the richest foods available. They're also extremely easy to cook or sneak into other dishes. For example, a can of artichoke hearts will easily fit into a dip or salad. Try to find ones in brine rather than oil as this will lower fat and calories and you can rinse a lot of the sodium away before using them.

Sweet Potatoes: While white potatoes are high in potassium they are usually so high in starch that they have a very low nutritional value. Sweet potatoes, on the other hand, have higher values of vitamin C and B6 as well as much needed fiber and calcium. The biggest benefit is that they are also one of the densest foods for vitamin A, a known antioxidant. Butternut squash has similar values and other squash varieties are also high in A and C vitamins.

Beans: Despite being considered as a "poor man's food" beans are rich in vitamins, minerals and antioxidants. Soybeans are also rich in zinc and selenium. Lentils have a high level of folate and zinc. One cup of red beans alone has a whopping 13,727 antioxidants in it. The fiber also found in beans has been linked to lower rates of colon cancer and lowered blood cholesterol as well which may reduce oxidative stress. Peanuts are technically in the same family as beans but we'll cover them under nuts for sanity's sake.

Sea Vegetables: Rich in flavinoids sea vegetables have a dense amount of bio-available nutrients. The algae we mentioned before has a natural anti-UV antioxidant and can be eaten directly. Sea vegetables are also rich in iodine and vanadium. Many antioxidant enzymes require vanadium to function properly. Another important reason to include sea vegetables in your diet is that the antioxidants found in them are either flavinoid or carotenoid based but have a unique structure. There have been some tenuous links between eating a diet including sea vegetables and a lowered risk for estrogen-related cancer.

Fish:

Rich in Omega-3's, fish is a healthy addition to any diet. It's strong anti-inflammatory properties rival those of antioxidants even if the fish itself does not actually have any. Tuna, salmon, sardines, trout, and herring are all rich in omega-3 fatty acids as well as being rich in vitamin D. Try and choose fresh fish over processed to avoid unnecessary free-radical intake.

Fruits

Grapes: The dark color of many foods is a great indication of rich antioxidants. Dark colored grapes are loaded with phytochemicals which are an antioxidant that may provide some protection against free radicals that cause cancer. Light colored grapes do still have antioxidants but are not as rich, they are also a good source of selenium and vitamin C. Anthocyanins are also known to be important for pre-menopausal women's health.

Blueberries: The same anthocyanins are also found in greater concentration in blueberries. However, blueberries are also known to have a blend of vitamins that strengthens the immune system as well as having antioxidants that lower inflammation and protect cells from damage.

Strawberries: Rich in vitamin C they are also high in a variety of minerals like folate, manganese, biotin, potassium, copper and iodine. Strawberry antioxidants have been studied for their anti-carcinogenic properties. They are also very bioavailable. When eating with blueberries and grapes strawberries have the highest composition of phenols of any fruit combination. 8 strawberries provide a higher amount of vitamin C than a whole orange!

Kiwi: People often forget that apples are not the only green fruit. Kiwis are rich in vitamins A and E which provides strong protection against free radicals. Kiwi fruit has also been linked to better heart health and can help lower cholesterol.

Açai: Considered to be a "hipster" food açai berries have gotten a lot of press recently because of their high antioxidant count. Essentially the açai berry has everything the blueberry has but in greater proportion. They are known to have a significant effect on cardiovascular and arterial health.

Grains

Whole grains are also rich in antioxidants. Research has shown that many whole grain cereals have large amounts of antioxidants, the problem is most of them are also supplemented. Polyphenols and fiber found in many whole grains have been shown to lower the risk of cancer and heart disease and have been found in comparable amounts to many fruits and vegetables. Wheat and oats have similar amounts of antioxidants to broccoli while corn has doubled that or apples. The problem with grains is that they are often highly processed with chemicals which add a side of free radicals with your antioxidants. Grains should be considered in moderation when trying to increase your antioxidant intake for this reason.

Herbs

Herbal remedies have been around for thousands of years, many people still swear by essential oils and herb tinctures. Many of our medicines are simply refined versions of the same compounds found in the original herbal remedies. Rather than eating the synthesized version go direct and use a selection of fresh herbs in your cooking. It will not only taste better but will boost the antioxidant content.

Oregano has the highest amount of antioxidants regardless of which type. It even has a higher antioxidant activity than many more well-known foods that are dense in vitamin E. Oregano has 42 times more activity than apples and even 4 times more than blueberries despite their being considered a "superfood". Rosemary, thyme, dill, and peppermint are also known to have high levels of antioxidants.

Tea and Coffee

Coffee: This is an instance where products are definitely not created equal. Though your morning cup of joe originally had antioxidants in much of the processing and roasting process that it goes through destroys any reasonable amount of antioxidants in it. Coffee in its rawest form is rich in hydrocinnamic acids and polyphenols which are both powerful antioxidants. These are also often only found in coffee and not in fruits or vegetables which makes coffee an essential for a varied antioxidant diet. Isn't that great news? Organic blends that are not too dark are best as the level of antioxidants decreases with the darkness of the coffee. It's estimated that the majority of western antioxidant intake actually comes from coffee.

Tea: With quite possibly thousands of varieties of tea it's difficult to say which are best. Tea contains epigallocatechin-3-gallate which is one of the most powerful antioxidants. It's been linked to weight loss, increased fat oxidation, lowering chances of macular degeneration, improved cholesterol and in the fight against atherosclerosis. Green tea Is considered to have the highest level of antioxidants but white tea, red tea and some of the more unusual like pu-erh have all been shown to have impressive amounts of antioxidants. When choosing a tea blend try and go for loose leaf and organic as this helps to cut down on processing and will also lower the risk of adding free-radicals into the blend. In fact, it's been shown that the most carcinogen and contaminants in tea are often found in the bag itself rather than the blend.

Nuts

Pecans, walnuts, hazelnuts are all excellent sources of antioxidants. Peanuts should be taken with advisement because although they are also rich in antioxidants they are often processed using radiation (a known cause of free radicals) and can also contain a mold spore that is a carcinogen. Organic and raw nuts are usually the best choices as there is little processing, meaning that the antioxidants are likely to be intact.

Conclusion

WHEN IT COMES TO THE FIGHT AGAINST AGING, cancer, and other diseases antioxidants pack a strong punch. Free radicals can wreak havoc on the body if left unchecked with oxidative stress being among one of the primary causes for over 60 different diseases.

In the fight against free radicals, there is no greater weapon than a diet rich in antioxidants. Supplements may help but they have also been shown to be ineffective against disease when compared to the real food version. Studies have shown that even though a diet rich in antioxidants may have some preventative powers actually consuming antioxidants once diagnosed with cancer can actually have the opposite effect.

Antioxidants found in foods often come in blends unavailable in supplements which is what makes them work so well as a preventative. While they may help slow down the aging process and improve your quality of life they are by no means a cure for the western diet. In fact, without having proper nutrition your body may have a level of oxidative stress that cannot be helped with supplements at all.

While choosing a diet based on a rainbow of foods can help improve your intake adding coffee and tea will do more. Not only are they calorie free (without additions like milk and sugar) but they pack a dense antioxidant amount. Many fruits and vegetables are high in antioxidants but surprisingly there are others like beans and grains which are just as important.

To maximize results from an antioxidant rich-diet don't forget to lower your sugar intake and exercise regularly. A diet rich in antioxidants is a prescription many of us need if we want to achieve optimum health.

Antioxidants might not be the magical key that many doctors promote them as but research has shown that they have definite health benefits.

www.ingramcontent.com/pod-product-compliance
Lightning Source LLC
Chambersburg PA
CBHW071315280526
45788CB00004B/1906